# A Survival Guide

## for
## Activity Professionals
### Second Edition

by Richelle N. Cunninghis, EdM, OTR/L

edited by Nancy DeBolt, BA, ACC

Published and distributed by

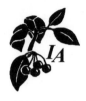

Idyll Arbor, Inc.

PO Box 720, Ravensdale, WA 98051 (425) 432-3231

*Library of Congress Cataloging in Publication Data*
Cunninghis, Richelle N., 1936-
    A survival guide for activity professionals / by Richelle N. Cunninghis : edited by Nancy DeBolt. – 2nd ed.
        p. cm.
    Includes bibliographical references.
    ISBN 1-882883-16-0
    1. Long-term care facilities—Recreational activities. 2. Recreational therapists—Vocational guidance. I. DeBolt, Nancy. II. Title.
RA999.R42C86  1997
362.1'6—dc21                                                  97-16966

ISBN  1-882883-16-0

# Contents

**Publisher's note:**

The term "activity professional" is used throughout this book. By "activity professional" we mean an individual who provides activity services to residents in health care including those who are (but, of course not limited to):

- Activity Assistant Certified
- Activity Consultant Certified
- Activity Director Certified
- Art Therapist
- Dance Therapist
- Horticultural Therapist
- Music Therapist
- Occupational Therapist
- Occupational Therapy Assistant
- Recreational Therapist, NCTRC Certified
- Social Worker

This book is also intended for students who are preparing to be activity professionals.

*Chapter 1*

# Introduction

Activity professionals are the new kids on the block. They were the last members of the health care team to become established and recognized. Although mentions of activity programs can be found dating back to the late 50's, it was really not until 1966 — with the establishment of the Medicare program — that actual guidelines were established. The first handbook for those who were then called "Activities Supervisors" was published by the Public Health Service in 1969. This was revised and expanded in 1978 under a new title, **Activities Coordinator's Guide**, accompanied by a price hike from $1 to $6. Activity professionals had arrived!

It seems to me that the time now has come to look at the occupation of the activity professional and think about the future. Is it going to expand and grow and, indeed, endure? The constant threat of government cutbacks and the ever-changing regulatory environment create a volatile atmosphere in the health care industry. Activity programs may be the victims of economic squeezes by government, corporations and individual facilities.

My feeling is that the whole field has reached yet another crossroads and there is a great need for activity professionals to take positive action now. Not only do they represent the newest specialty in health care, but are probably the least well-defined. Requirements vary from state to state, as do the amounts of job-specific education received. Few states require the in-depth professional training that is demanded in other disciplines. Professionalism, I believe, is the key to the survival of people who provide activities.

The purpose of this manual is to help you achieve that greater sense of professionalism — through information and training techniques. It will not attempt to duplicate what is available from other sources about the role and duties of activity professionals. Rather, it is an outline of the management skills that are necessary for all members of the health-care team adapted specifically to your needs as activity professionals.

Exactly what is meant by "professionalism?" Although there are many definitions, the one that is being used here refers to respect for yourself and your job and the ability to convey that feeling to everyone with whom you come in contact.

It begins with behaving as a "professional" on the job — with a demeanor that says, "I was hired to do a job, I plan to do it and I will do it well." That may sound obvious but, only too often activity professionals give an impression of being very uncertain of themselves and their position in the facility. If they feel that they may, indeed, have lower status, what can they expect others to think? It is important to act with the assurance of "being in charge," and not to continually ask for support or approval or for others to intercede on their behalf.

To do this you need to evaluate yourself with honesty. Take a long, hard look at yourself and what you think you bring to your job. Recognize both your strengths and your limitations and seek appropriate help for the latter. This is far preferable to struggling along and having others point out your shortcomings. People respect those who can say "I am not familiar with this," or "This is an area where I've never had any training. Could you help me?" If there is no one in the facility who can help, ask if you could have a short-term consultant or attend a course, workshop or seminar. In some cases it may even be worthwhile to pay for it yourself. But make sure you tell your administration what you are doing and why you are doing it.

All health care professionals take pride in updating their knowledge and skills. Activity professionals can be credentialled as an activity director certified (ADC), certified therapeutic recreation specialist (CTRS); occupational therapist registered (OTR) or certified occupational therapy assistant (COTA), for instance, and in order to retain those credentials must take part in ongoing educational opportunities.

An awareness of dressing as a professional is important. Many jeans-clad or mini-skirted activity professionals complain that no one takes them seriously. Look at the other staff members in your facility. How do they dress? What messages are they sending? There is nothing wrong with dressing appropriately and informally for certain activities, but the rest of the time you should look like a professional. Try uniforms or smocks if your work is too hard on your wardrobe, but make sure that they are clean and always fresh looking. Jewelry, make-up, shoes, etc. are all part of the picture and should be considered by you in forming your "image."

A telling aspect of professional behavior is to give and take credit appropriately. Pat others on the back when they deserve it (including members of your own department) and accept compliments from others. "Yes, it did turn out well, didn't it?" Too often people, in general, cannot handle compliments gracefully. So if you deserve praise, then, by all means, agree. On the other hand, don't be upset if you don't get credit for something you did. Be content to know you did it. After all, the residents were the beneficiaries in most cases and they usually are very appreciative.

A closely allied area is relationships with other staff members. This will be discussed later in greater depth, but it is important that you educate your colleagues every chance you get about the exact role you and your department play. Give in-services that will help familiarize them with this role; be prepared and make appropriate contributions at staff conferences and meetings. Be aware of the scope of your job, help define it for others and protect it from those who would like to take pieces of it away. Work on increasing your communication skills so that you can do these things effectively and in non-threatening ways.

Familiarize yourself with the regulations that may affect you as they pertain to your department and to the facility as a whole. If you are not given copies, request them. After all, you are being held responsible for the implementation of these regulations and, you will agree, that is tough to do if you have not seen them. If you request a copy of the regulations and it is not forthcoming, you might consider purchasing it yourself.

Evaluate your program, its place in the facility and your role in it periodically — from the view of an outsider. Where is the program going? What is being added? What will it look like a year from now? Five years? Most businesses and industries look at their status every year and set goals, objectives and plans for the coming year. This is something you should be doing, too. Nothing gets changed if provisions are not made for change. Approach it as you approach resident care plans. Assess where you are now and then ask yourself what problems you can identify and what changes you would like to make. For those that can be realistically implemented, set goals with time frames, consider budgetary limitations and outline the steps you are going to take to reach these goals. These could include such things as adding new programs, reaching more residents on a one-to-one basis, learning skills necessary to start a program in something like ceramics, buying new equipment, finding new sources of entertainment, increasing staff or starting or adding to volunteer programs. Remember, staff need to grow and enhance their skills or they and the program will stagnate.

And, finally, form groups and associations, both formal and informal, with other activity professionals. Start in your local area and identify training, legislative and professional concerns and needs. Share resources, problem-solving strategies and programs. Explore affiliation with regional or national groups whose aims may be the same as yours.

Look towards the future and establish your visibility as a professional now. One idea might be to provide speakers for other groups about the role that activity plays in long term care settings and adult day care centers. Hold conferences and meetings and invite prominent people and the press. The more publicity you can get, the better. It is important to educate the public, too. In fact, this should be considered part of the job for anyone who works with the elderly. The more you can promote the role and image of the activity professional as an important part of the team caring for the elderly, the better the future of that role will be.

Let us start by looking at how you can begin to "professionalize" your role within your own facility. Each of the following chapters will deal with one aspect of the job of activity professional. They will provide information on the skills necessary to increase your effectiveness in that particular area, beginning with establishing your territory and legitimate place within your facility.

## Chapter 2

# How to Define and Defend Your Turf

*Do you have a clear understanding of the responsibilities of the other departments in your facility?*

*Do they have a clear understanding of your department?*

*Do you understand all the requirements and limitations of your obligations and where and when it is appropriate for you to intervene?*

Before you can begin to think about defining and defending your turf, you must ask these questions and determine if you and the rest of your facility have the same ideas about which responsibilities belong to whom. Quite often grave misconceptions exist among departments about exactly what each is supposed to do. This is particularly true of the activity department. Many times there is great resentment toward activity professionals and their requests from those who think that they "have it easy" or "do nothing but play all day." So, how do you go about changing that?

Start with your job description. Read it thoroughly. If you don't have one, ask. There has to be one in the facility. (It is a requirement.) Actually, you shouldn't have taken the job without asking to see it. After you familiarize yourself with its contents — items included and not included — begin to question. "Why am I responsible for this duty if it isn't in my job description?" Or, "It says in my job description that this is a function of my department. Why is it being done by others?" There probably will be many things that are considered the responsibility of your department that are not included in the job description. Try to find out why. Some possible explanations may include:

**Tradition**: Your predecessor did it, so you are expected to do it. One simple example of this is an activity professional who used to go out and get a sandwich for lunch every day and bring it back to eat. She took orders from others and brought back their lunches as well. When she left the facility, her replacement was also expected to take lunch orders even though she brought her lunch with her every day and had no desire to go out.

**Expediency**: There is no one else to do it. It doesn't fit into anyone else's job description, so it must belong to the activity department. I am sure that all of you can provide your own examples for this one!

**Misunderstood boundaries**: Usually activity professionals have no one to blame for this one but themselves. The result is a loss of control — others decide what is appropriate for activity professionals to do or how they should do it. Examples include: allowing the nursing department to decide which residents should go to an activity, rather than providing them with a list that you have drawn up with the input of the interdisciplinary care team; or doing a lot of personal shopping for residents that really should be a function of the social services department.

**Ignorance**: This is a result of not being informed and not taking the trouble to find out. Many times activity professionals are doing jobs that they don't have to do, or others should do, simply because they don't know how to summon available help.

**Administrative request**: When considering tasks that you might not think appropriate, make sure you know who is making the request. Although a long shot, you sometimes may be able to convince your supervisor of the inappropriateness of such demands.

**Trading of services**: Often staff will help each other out when someone is short-handed. This is common practice and beneficial to all as long as the helping is not done by only one department and does not consistently interfere with its own operations.

After you have looked at your job carefully and identified those things that you think do or do not properly belong to you, decide which ones are really worth trying to change. Some may just be minor annoyances, while others may be very time consuming and causes of great stress.

Next, you have to consider risk. If you do take a position on some of these issues, what do you stand to lose? It could be your "nice guy" image or it could possibly be your job. (More likely the consequences will fall somewhere in between.) Are you willing to take that risk? Are the possible gains greater than the possible losses? Of course it is not always possible to know the answers exactly, but you should make an objective evaluation of the situation before taking any action.

That objective evaluation begins with prioritizing the issues you've discovered. Which is the most important to change? Which is the least? Work on one at a time and realize that redesigning your responsibilities to fit your job description may take sustained effort and some time.

For those issues you decide to tackle, choose your strategy very carefully. Remember, change is very difficult for everyone and most people are very resistant initially. Timing, approach and proper choice of words are crucial. Try to present your case so that it sounds like the change will be beneficial for all. For example, one approach that has proved effective in the situation of shopping for residents is to approach the social services department and apologize for having taken over some of its responsibilities. Say you were only trying to be helpful, didn't mean to overstep your bounds and would like to place the task back where it rightfully belongs. It's hard to resist an approach like that.

As for those things that you decide not to try to change, accept your own decision. You have explored them as issues and decided that they are not worth the effort or successful change for your department is unobtainable, so just add them to your job description and don't waste any more time with them.

Now that you have defined your turf — where your job ends and other jobs begin — how do you defend it? First, help the rest of the staff to understand this as well. Find out as much as possible about others and their jobs and never miss an opportunity to explain about yours. If you are challenged about why a particular resident doesn't go to activities, you might explain about initial assessments, residents' rights and the definition of activity that says that everything a resident does during his waking hours, except treatment, is considered activity. And tell them how that resident is, indeed, involved in activities. Share with others the criteria that you use to select residents for certain activities and why this one isn't suitable for Mrs. X while something else may be. If you are not asked to do in-service programs on activities, then try to get permission from the facility in-service director to do one. (There is a sample outline for an activity program inservice at the end of the chapter.) You might also ask if such programs couldn't be given by other departments as well, so that all the staff will have a better idea of each department's responsibility.

Never miss an opportunity to build bridges and clarify roles with other staff members. For example, if you are taking new residents, visitors or volunteers on a tour of the day program and you encounter other staff members, introduce them to your guests with a comment such as "This is Mrs. Smith. She is one of the people responsible for the great refreshments we have at our parties" or "You can always count on Mr. Jones here if you need something fixed right." It is a way of giving colleagues recognition, expressing thanks and telling them how much you appreciate their service to you and your department.

The following is a list of additional ideas that will help you define and defend your turf:

**Educate others formally and informally.** Do this every chance you get. Be sure to be prepared at interdisciplinary care meetings to specifically discuss resident participation and outcomes of involvement in activities.

**Establish your expertise.** You are the activity expert in your facility. You should make that clear to others who try to tell you how to do your job. Make it clear by assuming the responsibilities that go with the position and by doing the job well.

**Be professional.** There it is again. A professional is "one who knows." Demonstrate that you know your job through dress, manner and, above all, proper preparation. All have great bearing on how successful you are in establishing your territory.

**Resist attempts to reduce your status or authority.** Be firm, when appropriate, in dealings with other departments. Return (or better yet, call and ask others to return) residents who are brought to activities inappropriately because the floor staff can't stand their noise anymore. If you have requested chairs and tables be set up for a special event and find them piled up outside your door, don't move them. Call the department responsible, thank them for delivering them and ask them now to please send someone to set them up as they can't be used the way they are. (One way to avoid this is to send a memo that includes a sample of the way that you want the room set up so there can be no misunderstanding.) Make it clear that under ordinary circumstances, you do not expect to do others' jobs or ask them to do yours.

**Keep careful records.** You need records not only on residents, programs and budget, but on your own use of time. If you can justify your time, it may help to prevent you from acquiring additional jobs that you can't handle. If not, make this suggestion to your administrator: "I would be glad to add that to my duties. Please look at my schedule and help me decide what I should eliminate to make room for it?"

**Be aware of the needs and schedules of other departments.** Try to take these into account when involving them in programming. For example, know how much time the dietary department requires to order special foods, when the housekeeping department regularly schedules the waxing of the activity room floor or when the nursing department might be short-handed because of a scheduled in-service or the podiatrist's visit.

**Identify the power structure in your facility.** Then work within it. Sometimes the people who actually make the decisions and have the most power are not those who have the most visibility. Take a good look at the politics and chain-of-command and make sure that you are following the rules that are set down.

**Apply a magic formula to everything you are told.** Always ask:

- Who said so?
- What did s/he say, exactly?
- How do you know? (What is your source of information?)

These are particularly helpful in situations where you are told, "You are not allowed to do that!" or "This is the way we do it around here." By asking these questions, you often discover that there is no authority for these statements. They are just someone's misconception of what is permissible.

**Use your skills of effective communication.** It is necessary for everyone to remember that all of you are there for the same purpose — to serve the residents. Unfortunately, experience has shown us that disputes over turf often interfere with effective resident care.

# Sample Activities Inservice

I.  What things are important to you?

    A. List 3 things you like to do in your spare time: hobbies, leisure activities, etc.

    B. Imagine that you were 30-40 years older and in a nursing home. Will you still find the same things important? Will you still be able to do them? How will you have to change them?

    C. Share feelings with others. This can be done in small groups or the entire group.

II. This is what activity programs the people we serve are all about:

    A. They always start with an identification of needs, interests and what is important to each individual.

    B. The goal of activity programming is to create and support an enriched environment for quality living which relates to each individual's life style.

    C. The definition that is used for "activity" is anything a person does during his waking hours that is not treatment.

        1. Ask "What does that include?" (List)

        2. Ask "How can we do a better job in this facility to help maintain previous roles of our residents, such as consumer, homemaker, citizen, worker?

        3. Activities must be integrated into daily life, not thought of as a separate entity.

III. Role of other staff in activities

    A. Others, particularly certified nursing assistants, are in position to see and hear things that activity professionals often are not.

        1. Ask that they pass on anything that might impact participation: changes in condition or behavior.

        2. Are there any suggestions that might improve the total program or the individualized program of particular residents?

        3. Can they add anything that would help you and your department, such as having residents ready on time, encouraging attendance, not bringing anyone that is not requested, help in escorting to and from activities, etc.

    B. How can activity professionals make their job easier?

    C. What would they like to see done differently?

*Chapter Three*

# How to Manage Time More Effectively

*Do you recognize this scene? In the morning as she comes in the door, the activity professional stops at the nursing station to socialize and talk about last night's date or fight with her husband, starts to change the information on the reality orientation board, realizes she is out of a letter that she needs, goes to find it, is stopped by a resident who never had her mail read to her yesterday, reads the mail, picks up her embroidery to match the thread, helps another who can't reach something in her closet, is called to the telephone, tries to find her appointment book to check a date for entertainment, realizes she has missed a meeting, etc., etc. and then wonders where the morning went?*

If you can relate to this, you probably need some help managing of your time through an introduction to time management techniques.

It is good to begin with the assumption that things are not going to get better next week, nor after Christmas, after the open house, after inspection, after...! That attitude alone probably prevents many people from getting started on a successful time management program. The goals of a time management program are to get you to set objectives, assign priorities, overcome indecision and conquer chronic worry and procrastination. But remember, time management techniques are only tools. They can't do the job for you, but they certainly can make the job easier.

Although many of us know the right things to do, we aren't motivated to do them. Information is useless if it isn't utilized. You can't become organized by reading a book on techniques!

The first questions you have to ask yourself are

- What is the purpose of my job?
- Why does it exist?
- What are the major activities or tasks that I must perform to accomplish the purpose of my job?

No one understands your job and your priorities better than you do. There are no single "right" answers, even for two activity professionals in similar situations.

Write a list of all the tasks and activities that make up your job. Then ask yourself, for each one, "What would happen if I didn't do it?" Discard all those items that get an answer of "nothing." Then look at the rest and divide them into categories.

1. Establish priorities by dividing tasks into those which must be done today and those which can be put off until tomorrow.

2. Determine what must be done by you or what can be delegated to someone else. (Don't worry about who the someone else might be at this point. We will come back to that later.)

3. Break overwhelming tasks into manageable pieces (e.g., divide 60 residents progress notes required every 3 months into 20 per month, which can be reduced to five a week or one a day).

4. Refine your list. Even things that can be put off now can't be put off indefinitely, so set deadlines for when they must be done. (Methods will be introduced later that will aid in doing this.)

5. Identify time wasters. You have identified where your time should be going, now look at where it actually is going.

## *Reasons People Waste Time*

Before you look specifically at how you waste time, take a minute to consider why you mismanage time. Do you recognize what you are getting from the things that you do? Sometimes it is easier to change habits if you know why you do them. And sometimes you must accept that there are certain things you don't want to change because the rewards are too great. These considerations will just have to be built into your time management plan.

Many people waste time to get attention. They are constantly operating in a crisis situation and make sure that everyone is aware of how much they have to do and how little time there is to do it. Others enjoy the excitement and stimulation of crisis management, which is working under the pressure of leaving everything to the last minute. This is often a life-long pattern and reflects a struggle against structure as well as a need for constant challenge.

There are those who resist change by refusing to get anything completed. They avoid working with others or avoid the risk of failure (or success) by not coping. Some people fear they really are not capable or conversely, that they may be ridiculed for doing "too good" a job.

Others shirk personal responsibility, avoid unpleasant tasks, try to gain a sense of power or control or try to look busy all the time as sole justification for their job. Some people have an overriding need for perfection. They are never satisfied that a task is completed right and consequently continue to work on something after it is good enough, still feeling, perhaps, that they should do even better!

Many of us have a need to be considered a "friend to the world," a general all-around "good guy," a constant victim of other people and situations or always "in the know about what goes on around here." These are the people who spend time in socializing, counseling and gossiping, anything but the provision of activity programming!

Procrastination, inability to say "no," personal disorganization, indecision and lack of use of support personnel can be wasteful as well. Any or all of these lead to wasting time — time that should go to the primary functions of your job.

## Time Wasters

Time wasters come in all shapes and forms. Let's look at some of the most common ones and the sources from which they spring.

**The Telephone** Problems here are often caused by:

- enjoyment of socialization
- desire to be available, involved, informed
- feelings of importance when receiving calls
- lack of delegation or screening of calls
- not having facts available or an agenda of items to be discussed
- fear of offending
- lack of self-discipline
- inability to terminate conversations

**Visitors** These can be residents, volunteers, family members or other staff members, but the problems are still the same:

- all of those listed under telephone
- requiring others to check with you excessively
- open-door policy
- facility protocol and precedence
- confused responsibilities
- unrealistic conception of time requirements

**Meetings** Often these are beyond your control and your presence is required (or is it?). But they may suffer from:

- a lack of purpose
- a lack of agenda or the ability to adhere to it
- being held in the wrong place and/or at the wrong time
- too many people present
- inadequate notice resulting in poor participation
- not starting and/or ending on time
- socializing
- interruptions
- indecision
- lack of follow-through

**Crisis Development** Crises can be a result of:

- lack of planning
- lack of awareness that a situation is building up
- failure to anticipate realistically
- attempting too much
- over-reacting to all situations
- procrastination
- not doing the job right the first time
- inaccurate priorities
- responding to wrong information

**Failure to Delegate Successfully** This is one of the major tenets of time management. It is often not accomplished because of:

- insecurity or fear of failure
- lack of confidence in staff
- need to involve yourself in everything
- giving incomplete or unclear instructions
- envy of subordinate's ability
- feeling that you can do the job better and faster
- being more comfortable doing than managing
- failure to establish controls or over-controlling
- lack of follow-up
- being understaffed or having overworked subordinates
- not having anyone to whom to delegate

**Inability to Say "No"** This is a problem for everyone at one time or another because of our:

- not being aware that this is a problem
- desire to help people
- desire to win approval and acceptance
- fear of offending
- fear of losing job

- being very capable and efficient
- false sense of obligation
- insecurity or low self-esteem
- guilt feelings
- not assessing consequences
- finding it easier to say "yes"
- lack of excuses
- fear of retaliation
- desire to put other in our debt
- losing sight of our own objectives and priorities
- inability to cope with others who refuse to accept responsibility

**Lack of Self-Discipline** It can be difficult to admit, but it's often a problem because of our:

- lack of planning
- lack of objectives or standards
- lack of priorities
- not setting deadlines
- doing what we like, not what we should
- postponing unpleasant or difficult tasks
- not following up
- not utilizing available resources
- being lazy
- lack of awareness of the problem
- lack of interest or motivation
- inability to say "no"
- drifting into trivia
- cluttered desk and workspace
- leaving tasks unfinished
- carelessness
- daydreaming
- fatigue, poor health or personal problems
- procrastination
- poor work habits

- undisciplined supervisor or organization
- switching tasks and priorities mid-stream
- acceptance of unwarranted interruptions

To sum up, most time wasters fall into five major categories:

1. Inability to assert yourself to make sure you are doing the work you need to do.
2. Failure to delegate which makes you work below your level of capabilities. If it can be done by someone else, it should be.
3. Toleration of too many interruptions.
4. Avoidance of big or undesirable tasks by wasting time on little pleasant ones.
5. Improper preparation or working without a plan.

The last is perhaps, the most serious. For not only does it get you off the track, make you look bad and cause repetition but, by a ripple effect, it causes delays for other people. Incidentally, while going through this process, you might ask yourself how you interfere with other departments. Do *you* often waste the time of *other* staff members?

There is one final question to ask yourself about time wasters, "Who controls my time?" Although there may be things that you see as being a waste of your time, if your supervisor does not and you cannot convince him/her otherwise, then build it into your schedule. Don't multiply the effect by sulking, griping or otherwise reacting negatively. Accept those things you cannot change, but be aware of the signals that you are sending out to others that might be saying that your time is not a priority. Signals that say you are always available invite people to interfere with your attempts to plan and manage your time.

# Strategies for Dealing with Time Wasters

Let's look at some of the identified time wasters and see if there aren't some ways to minimize them.

**Meetings** Before calling or attending any meetings, ask yourself these questions:

- Is my presence necessary?
- Are all these people necessary?
- Does this really require a formal meeting? (Or a regularly scheduled meeting?)
- Is there a written agenda for the meeting?
- Am I prepared?
- Are there specific starting and stopping times?
- Is the room so comfortable that people are going to stay?

Using these guidelines, it is fairly easy to make sure that you are prepared, that attempts are made to stay with the agenda and to leave at the appointed hour with a statement such as "I have an activity scheduled now because I expected that the meeting would be over as planned." This might even give others the needed push to do the same thing.

**People** The most effective way to deal with interruptions by staff, families, visitors or residents is to set limits. Start by saying something like "I can only give you five minutes." Or, "I can't talk to you now. I usually set aside time between 4:00 and 4:30 for conferences. Could I see you then?" Or stand up when someone comes in and say "I'm sorry, but I was just on my way to ..." And stick to the limits that you set!

If necessary, isolate yourself. Put a "Do Not Disturb" sign on the door or find a place that does not have too much traffic. Avoid places where people go to smoke, use the telephone, buy sodas, etc.

**The Telephone** Similar techniques work here. If possible, get the switchboard to hold your calls and tell people you will receive and/or return calls between certain designated hours. Install an answering machine, Get right to the heart of the matter and ask people why they are calling, with a minimum of social chatter. Tell them you are extremely busy today.

If you have trouble terminating conversations, try phrases like "Before I let you go ..." or "I don't want to take any more of your time." If it is more comfortable, use phrases such as these: "I must go because someone is waiting," "I have another phone call" or "It's time for an activity," etc.

**Say "No"** This one might be a little tougher because it is probably a life-long pattern to say "Yes." By your agreeing to a task, even a small one, outside the scope of your job, you may make friends of other staff members, but you put pressure on yourself to accomplish your job responsibilities in less time. Therefore, these gifts of your time may become time wasters. The best advice is to just say "No" instead. Don't get trapped into giving a lot of excuses. Just say "No, I can't" and walk on. If it is necessary to give reasons, be truthful. "I don't really want to," "I don't think it's part of my job" or "I just don't have the time." And, most importantly, don't waste time feeling guilty. You are probably doing more than you should in the first place!

Also learn to say "No" to yourself. Establish acceptable levels of performance for what you do and stop when they are reached. Enough is enough!

**Organize Your Desk and Workspace** First, be sure that you have a work center for yourself with a desk, files, etc. And then keep it clean. Try to have a designated place for everything and be sure that you (and everyone else) return things immediately after using them to these designated places.

If your desk is a pile of clutter, start by going through it and separating things into three piles.

1. *Important work:* tackle these by going through one by one immediately.

2. *To be delegated:* pass on to the proper person.

3. *Unimportant:* put or, better yet, throw it away. (It will probably stay there until it is too late to do anything else with it anyway!)

If tasks in the first group are very large, divide them into manageable pieces. Set priorities and deadlines for each part and utilize a "tickle file," a system in which a calendar or card file is used to list jobs to be done on each day. You use it by planning ahead and filling in the appropriate tasks on the appropriate days. For example, if you know you have a report that is due for your administrator by the end of the month, you might make a note on the 23rd to start working on the report. If you are planning a special event, determine the steps and time-frames required to choose the date, contact entertainment, notify dietary, etc. and enter them in the right places. Using this method, you should never be caught short at the last minute trying to get everything done, as long as you remember to enter the data and look at the tickle file every day!

Don't reinvent the wheel. If something works, save it so you can use it again. Have activity plans written up so you know exactly what you need and how to run each activity. (See the sample on the next page.) After each special event or even things like monthly birthday parties, review the procedures and decide how long each step needed. Then write it down in a permanent file and, when appropriate, enter it in your tickle file. Devise standard forms so that the information can easily be filled in each time. Perhaps one memo form could be utilized, sent to each department involved, filled out once and duplicated. (A sample form is shown on the second following page.)

## *Activity Plan*

Title _____

Purpose _____

Participants (group size, sex, physical/mental requirements)

_____

_____

Equipment and Supplies _____

_____

Room Set-Up _____

_____

Personnel Requested _____

_____

Precautions and Special Considerations _____

_____

_____

Identified Problems and Solutions_____

_____

_____

Preparation Time _____

Activity Steps

| What | When | Who |
|------|------|-----|
| | | |
| | | |
| | | |
| | | |
| | | |
| | | |
| | | |
| | | |
| | | |

Prepared By _____Date_____

# *Special Event Request Form*

Title of Event _____

Purpose _____
_____

Date _____ Time Start_____ End _____

Number of People _____ Location _____

Food Required _____
_____

Supplies Required _____
_____

Room Set-Up _____
_____

Diagram of Set-Up




Personnel Requested _____
_____
_____

Special Needs_____
_____
_____

Prepared By _____Date_____

**Communication** A big part of your time is spent in communicating with the public, volunteers, families, other staff, as well as with residents. As you've noted, this, too, can be a time trap. If you spend time being a messenger or explaining the same things over and over again to a variety of people, you are not communicating *or* managing time effectively.

Use memos whenever possible. Make sure that you always keep a copy of every memo you send. Send copies of the monthly calendar to all concerned with important information included. Write up explanations of any program or idea that you want to implement and send out copies to volunteers, staff, residents or department heads who may be involved in its implementation.

One of the cardinal rules of time management is never to handle the same piece of paper twice. Try to get in the habit of going through your mail and taking care of it right away. Throw away most of it. Reply on the same sheet if it can be done conveniently or file it in the proper place. These same steps should be taken with any piece of paper that comes across your desk.

**General Time Savers** Determine which are your hours of peak efficiency and try to do the hardest tasks during the time when you are at your best. Consolidate related tasks and try to do them all at one time, either by location or equipment or time required.

Use spare moments effectively to go through catalogues, catch up on reading materials, write memos or make plans. Reschedule activities where you are running into interference. For example, one activity professional found that the best time for her to do her documentation was while the residents

31

were at dinner. She altered her working hours to accommodate this block of useful time.

Be realistic about how long a task is going to take when planning. Don't underestimate the time needed because almost everything takes longer than you think it will. Also don't schedule so tightly that you do not allow time for preparation and for getting from one place to another. One facility divided its morning calendar into half-hour reality classes, with a new one starting at the same time that the previous one ended. This, of course, did not allow for transportation of residents or for staff to catch its breath. Be realistic when doing planning. Don't expect yourself or your employees to work at full speed all the time.

## Delegating Work

Several mentions have been made of the delegation of tasks and responsibilities. You must be aware of how vital this principle is. When you don't delegate, you:

- deny subordinates the opportunity for learning and growth
- cheat yourself of the time to do more important and creative things
- deprive the facility and residents of your best work
- rob your family by working when you could be spending time with them

There are many reasons accepted for not delegating. The solutions for most of them are obvious, but let's look at the last one — not having anyone to delegate to. Even if you are the only activity professional in the facility, there are people available who can help you. How about residents, volunteers, family members or other staff? In some facilities the receptionist or switchboard operator is willing to help the activity department when s/he is not busy. Others use secretarial staff or ward clerks in appropriate functions. Sometimes it is necessary to look very closely at tasks and see what could be done by others. And often it is the parts that are the most time-consuming that are the best candidates for delegation.

A word of caution, however. Although you should, whenever possible, delegate tasks that do not need your personal attention, make certain that you allow time to oversee or review the work that you have delegated. (There will be further discussion of the topic of delegation in the chapter on supervision.)

## *Action Plan*

Many ideas have been given here for better use of time. In addition, it is necessary to actually make a plan. This is almost identical to the way that you do resident documentation. Much of this chapter has concerned itself with assessment and problem identification. The next step is to set goals, both long- and short-term, with priorities and deadlines. Then come the plans. These can include daily "to-do" lists, your tickle file, delegation plans and allocation of specific blocks of time for each item. The priority should be to accomplish the job that needs to be done with a minimum of stress for all involved.

When you mismanage your time, ask yourself, "What is this day for?" "What is the best use of my time right now?" And most importantly, remember that time management is not a one-time thing. It must be kept up on a continuing basis. The majority of people find that once they begin to take charge of time and to manage their job life effectively, it is the only way they care to operate. Time management has become second nature.

*Chapter 4*

# How to Be an Effective Supervisor

*Your facility has been expanding and when the new wing opens, two new activity assistants are to be added to the staff. You have just been informed that you are responsible for hiring and supervising these two people. Where do you start?*

This is a good opportunity to look at exactly what is required of activity professionals in your facility. List all the duties you can think of that go with the job. Then, go over the list and put a check next to those that you do well. The ones that remain will give you a pretty good idea of the characteristics to look for in your new assistants. That doesn't mean that you will get to keep all those things you do well or that your new people will have to do everything else, but this technique helps to provide a balance of skills and abilities in the department. For example, you may not be particularly skilled in crafts or talented in music or you prefer one-to-one relationships because you are uncomfortable leading large group activities. Trying to fill these gaps might be wise. Certainly writing skills and the ability to relate well to people who are older are standard skills for all activity professionals.

Then begins the interview and evaluation process. Try to hire the best available people. Don't view capable people as a threat, but rather as a means of increasing the effectiveness of your department — a means of giving better resident care and making your job more productive.

Good training is essential to the success of your new employees. Their orientation program should include an introduction to the philosophy, history and physical layout of the facility, as well as to other staff members and their functions. They should be provided with appropriate general information about aging, disease processes and, of course, the duties of the job itself.

Identify for them the goals of your department within the organization and those you personally are trying to achieve. Make every effort to find out what they want from this job. Encourage them to set goals for themselves and to indicate how you might help them reach these goals.

It is important that those you are going to supervise understand clearly the work that is expected of them, including its quality and quantity. And they should have input into setting these standards as all people need to feel that they have some influence in making the decisions which affect them.

Don't make assumptions about how others are going to think, feel or react; rather encourage them to tell you. Indicate that you are available for guidance and supervision and do not expect them to perform at one hundred percent right away. Tell them they will be encouraged to grow with the job and will be given opportunities to assume greater responsibilities when they are ready. And you may also want to assure them that you will make every effort to provide new challenges and stimulation so they will not become bored with the routine tasks that they also will be required to do.

# What Does A Supervisor Do?

Before you can become an effective supervisor, you need to know the full scope of the role — just what is a supervisor and what will be expected of you. For the sake of simplicity, let us divide the responsibilities into two major components:

1. Management Ability or Administrative Skills  *Tasks*
2. Leadership or People-Handling Skills  *Human Relations*

One has to realize, of course, that it is not always possible to completely separate the two. In fact, on occasion they may even conflict.

But, for now, let's start with management ability. This refers to the responsibility you have to the organization of which you are a part. You are the liaison between those above and those below you. You are the management person that your employees deal with every day. This part of your job includes the supervisory skills of planning and organizing.

**Planning** involves determining the most effective means of accomplishing the work of the department. Your job is to:

- *Identify* the main goals and objectives as prescribed by the administration, keeping in mind that the well-being of the residents is the primary goal of every department within the facility and the main determinant of all other goals.

37

- *Decide* the most effective means of reaching the goals and objectives that have been identified, including additional skills and training that may be required.

Not only must you assess your department in terms of these goals, but you and your staff must determine what is yet to be accomplished. Then you must decide the best way to do that by formulating goals and plans. These steps must be completed or no other part of the supervisory process can follow.

**Organizing** involves distribution of work and assignment of job duties. These include scheduling of work assignments, coordination of programs, development and implementation of policies and procedures and setting the tone for the department. It also requires interrelationships with other departments for everyone's mutual benefit.

**Leadership skills** include the functions of employee development, motivation and direction. Both leadership and management components involve the function of *evaluation*, that is, assessment of how well the actual work is being accomplished compared to how it was planned. In most cases, this last function is the one for which the supervisor is totally responsible. As a supervisor, if things are not going as they should, it is up to you to determine why and then do something about it.

**Employee development** refers to the functions of selecting and training employees. The supervisor is responsible for measuring their performance and as previously indicated, providing opportunities for advancement and professional development.

**Motivation and direction** involve guiding, teaching and leading. Not only do they entail issuing instructions and

38

assignments but, perhaps more importantly, motivating each employee to work willingly and enthusiastically toward the department's goals. These tasks probably take more of a supervisor's time than any of the others and are often the most difficult to master. Let's look at the skills needed to perform these functions.

## Characteristics of A Good Supervisor

The characteristics of a good supervisor listed below are qualities emphasized in books, workshops, conversations and experiences. Certainly it is unrealistic to expect anyone to possess all these characteristics. But use the items on the list as guidelines and perhaps they will help you to enhance your capabilities. Good supervisors are

- committed to further personal growth, their own and others
- willing to seek advice and take it, if valid
- ready to give credit where due and accept criticism if justified
- organizationally sophisticated; they understand the system and means of working within it, its politics and power people
- aware of when it is important to challenge and when it is better to let things go
- able to speak, write and listen effectively
- knowledgeable about what motivates people to learn and perform; able to provide meaningful incentives
- aware of the importance of morale and, therefore, do not encourage or allow constant griping
- willing to relinquish control when it is good for the organization, but do not give power away to others

- able to analyze, assign and carry through on necessary tasks
- respectful of themselves and others
- accessible to employees; not isolated
- self-reliant and not afraid to make decisions because they might be the wrong ones
- willing to delegate and utilize available skills and resources, but also to pitch in and help when necessary
- aware of their role in the total organization and the chain of command
- willing to assume responsibility and lead, recognizing that authority and responsibility go together
- unwilling to take themselves too seriously and use humor liberally
- flexible, honest, discreet
- able to create an environment where people feel safe to contribute ideas and suggestions and where they don't feel threatened, but challenged
- willing to decrease uncertainty and anxiety by getting answers and decreasing unknowns whenever possible
- dedicated to making sure that everybody understands exactly what is expected of them
- consistent, supportive, objective and enthusiastic
- able to establish priorities and put first things first
- willing to look at themselves objectively, admit shortcomings and attempt to do something about their weaknesses
- able to bring out the best in others
- fair-minded so that they do not believe all they hear and when in doubt, check it out
- professional and proud of it

# The Function of Delegating

The main role of a supervisor is to define the common purpose of the department and help all staff members work toward the accomplishment of that purpose. Some try to do everything themselves and usually fail because they can't. You are not a leader when you are doing all the work. You have the responsibility for the common purpose and your employees should provide the action. Success is getting things done through your people, by learning to delegate.

Successful delegation includes three main steps:

1. Assign work and duties
2. Grant authority to use available resources and take all necessary actions to accomplish the task
3. Create responsibility to perform tasks satisfactorily

Assigning work involves matching task requirements to available skills and resources. Be aware of those things that can be done by others and, specifically, who the best people are to do them. Communicate in clear terms the exact task and when it should be completed. Though it means telling others *what* to do, it does not include telling them *how* to do it. Don't inhibit creativity and individual initiative.

Grant authority to the staff member to make decisions and act within predetermined limits in order to accomplish the tasks. If your employees have to check with you every step of the way, you might as well do it yourself in the first place.

Create responsibility for the outcome of the work. Everyone should be involved in the selection of appropriate tasks, solicitation of ideas and understand what is expected of them.

Then they can be held accountable for the work itself. However, keep in mind that you, as supervisor, remain ultimately accountable and always have the final responsibility. Therefore, much of your success depends on how well you help your employees recognize and meet their obligations.

Despite the importance of successful delegation, it is equally important to know which things are not appropriate for delegation. Some tasks are the duty of the supervisor and therefore must properly be done only by you. These include:

**Planning:** decide the goals to be implemented and in which order and by whom. It is appropriate to involve the whole department in discussion of these goals, but final decisions and authority remain with you.

**Personnel concerns:** hiring, firing, work assignments, evaluations and conflict resolutions.

**Creation of a work environment** in which the employees feel comfortable, challenged and appreciated.

# *Feedback and Constructive Criticism*

One last supervisory function that is worthy of special consideration is that of giving feedback and constructive criticism. A big part of your job as supervisor entails continuous appraisal of workers' performances. Appraisal involves the evaluation of such things as cooperation, dependability, output, willingness to learn, appearance, use and upkeep of materials and supplies, judgment, safety procedures, initiative, knowledge of the job, attitudes, etc.

Appraisal is a means of providing objective information about performance and skill levels, weaknesses and strengths.

When giving feedback and constructive criticism, it is necessary to assure that the recipient understands what you are saying, is ready and willing to accept it and is able to do something about it if s/he chooses. Keeping this in mind, there are generally accepted criteria for giving useful feedback. It should be

- intended to help the recipient
- given directly and based on a trusting relationship
- done promptly after observed behavior
- descriptive of the person's action and the effect it created
- non-threatening and non-judgmental
- focused on behavior and not the person
- specific with good, recent examples
- focused on strengths as well as weaknesses
- inclusive of only changeable behavior, such as habits and not physical characteristics
- limited to no more than the person can handle at one time
- given at a time of receiver readiness
- presented to allow time for discussion
- *always* done in private, when negative. Preferably in public if positive.

There are many methods of giving feedback from which to choose. The most obvious one is the verbal conference. If this is the one you choose, approach the conversation carefully. Try to start with praise and honest appreciation and ask questions, rather than using statements. "What is interfering with your getting this done?" "Do you feel you are having a problem with ...?" Tell them how their behavior affects you. "I am having a problem with ..." or "I get the feeling that ..." Indicate that you need their help in solving the problem. Don't use sarcasm, kidding or labeling.

Another possibility is to use one of a variety of projection techniques. Ask the person how someone else might interpret a particular situation, what s/he thinks a state surveyor might understand this to mean or does s/he think that other staff members might see something the same way that s/he did? Suggest that the person put himself/herself in the place of a resident and try to identify how s/he would feel. By projecting themselves into the position of someone else and seeing it through other eyes, people are often able to pick up on their mistakes and correct them without anything else having to be said.

Modeling is another way to give feedback. Let them watch you interview a resident, write a plan, lead a group. Then discuss the situation with them — what they saw, what was right, what could be improved, how they might have done it differently. A variation on this is to role play with them and try to lead them around the pitfalls that they usually experience.

Field visits to other facilities or departments might provide insights as might attending in-services or educational programs that cover some of the problems they are having. Sometimes hearing problems discussed in a non-specific group situation is sufficient to spur change.

It is important not only to evaluate your employees, but to periodically look at yourself in the same fashion. Analyze your own performance critically and identify your strengths and weaknesses. Try to determine how your supervisor sees you. Are there areas where you should be doing more, need additional training or feel changes could be made? Develop some plans as to how you might implement change in these areas and discuss them with your supervisor *before* s/he calls them to your attention.

And if you are the recipient of constructive criticism, try to be open-minded and not defensive. Make sure that you understand what is being said to you, perhaps giving examples and asking if that is the sort of thing that is meant. And then make some suggestions as to how you might go about rectifying the identified problems. Thank him/her for bringing them to your attention so quickly and giving you an opportunity to correct them before they became more serious. Remember that all of us have to learn to take constructive criticism as well as give it and just as this is a function you must perform for your employees, so must your supervisor do it for you.

## Why Supervisors Fail

Before leaving this subject, let's take a look at why some people never make effective supervisors. Although there is no right or wrong way to supervise or style of leadership, there are criteria that are almost imperative and others that are almost equally important not to do. Just as a list was provided for characteristics that are desirable, here is one for the things to avoid. Many supervisors fail because they:

- lack professionalism, consideration and respect for themselves and others
- are very secretive about their jobs and do not share even unimportant things with others in their department
- are unwilling or unable to delegate work
- are negative, inflexible and discourage input from others
- do not set goals, create vague goals or do not follow through

- isolate themselves, are unaware of what is actually going on in their department and are not available when their staff needs them
- have no great desire to lead, don't like giving orders and allow others to take over responsibilities
- want to be liked, continue to be "one of the gang" and don't want to pull rank
- are overly impressed with their position and alienate those they work with
- feel threatened by the ability of others
- are afraid to make decisions because they may be incorrect
- never admit to being wrong or having made mistakes and try to put the blame on others
- stifle initiative and creativity in others

People are often promoted to the rank of supervisor without any prior training or experience. The skills that are necessary to be a good activity professional are not the same as those required for supervision. Do not expect to know how to supervise right away. Every new job takes time to learn, particularly one that is dependent on other people. Effective supervisory skills come through practice and if you are not properly prepared, you owe it to yourself to build the skills that you need. Read, take courses, observe others. Expect to make mistakes while learning the job. The important thing is to learn from them. And, most of all, don't be too hard on yourself!

## Chapter 5

# How to Make Decisions and Solve Problems

*Do you ever have 27 evaluations that need to be done by tomorrow morning?*

*Is there one staff person who drives you up a wall because she always has something to say — no matter how busy you are?*

In your job, as well as in your everyday life, problems constantly arise. This is normal and is to be expected. In fact, just try to imagine how dull life would be without any problems!

But how do you face these problems? Evaluate them? Make decisions about the right course of action to take? Or, when to act or not to act? Whether problems are related to residents, staff, supervisors, volunteers or other persons or situations, the same decision-making methods can be utilized.

Ignoring problems or procrastinating in making decisions causes anxiety and stress, not only for you, but for those around you as well. It can also lead to loss of morale, opportunities and resources. And, in most cases, the problems do not go away. They remain to be dealt with. When faced with decisions, a useful maxim to remember is that the same amount of time will go by if you take action or if you don't. But in the latter case, you will have nothing to show for it.

Often decisions are avoided because people do not have the experience to recognize their options and to choose between them. In fact, the best solutions may be a combination of these options rather than an either/or situation.

As is the case with all the skills discussed in this manual, decision-making and problem-solving require practice. The more experience you get, the easier it becomes. The methods suggested here may seem unnecessarily long and complex, but it is suggested that you do not eliminate any of the steps the first few times you go through the process. After that, you will probably find it becomes automatic and you will be able to adapt it to your own way of doing things.

## *Steps in Problem-Solving*

There are many different approaches to problem-solving. All start, however, with a comparison of "what is" to "what should be" and an identification of what is needed to get there. In other words, problem-solving is finding the ways to change a current undesirable situation into a desired one. This includes several steps:

1. Identify the apparent problem
2. Outline possible causes and reactions
3. Set goals and analyze alternatives
4. Decide on a course of action
5. Evaluate results

# Problem Identification

Accurately identifying the problem is the most important and, often, the most difficult part of the process. Most situations are not problematical in themselves, but our reactions and responses make them so. For example, if you dislike paperwork, that is not really a problem. But, if you don't get it done on time, do a poor job or make everyone around you miserable, that's a problem!

Sometimes just looking at situations in those terms provides insights. It is often possible to see that the real problems are the result of inappropriate reactions or solutions and not the situations themselves.

It is also helpful to realize that situations that are problems for one person may not problems for another. So part of the process of identification is to ask "For whom is it a problem?" If someone has a habit that irritates you, whose problem is it? Can you realistically expect him/her to change or is it up to you to do something? Again, it is the reaction that is the problem, not the situation itself. Therefore, before going on to the next steps in this process make sure that you have defined and stated the problem correctly.

> "I put off doing my documentation to the last minute and then do a poor job because I am rushed."

What is the primary problem here — the documentation, the procrastination or the quality of the work?

> "I get upset when Jane wastes my time talking about silly things that don't interest me."

Is the problem the conversation or the response? If your problem involves other people, do not expect them to change unless they perceive their behavior as a problem to them. This is an important point because often others are completely unaware that their actions are causing a reaction in us. It is definitely our problem and not theirs! So, as you can see, it is necessary to identify the problem correctly before you can even begin to think of solutions.

## *Causes and Reactions*

After identifying the problem, look at it objectively and ask yourself:

- Is it my problem?
- Is it really any of my business?
- Am I doing something to help reinforce it?
- Are my reactions the real problem?
- Why do I react the way I do?
- Are there other possible ways of looking at the situation?
- Could it be due to poor communication, lack of knowledge, personality conflict or the structure of my organization?

Perhaps you will be able to see more clearly now that it isn't Jane's conversation that is the problem, but your resentment of her wasting your time or, perhaps, your anger because you have more to do than she has.

Why do you put off documentation? Is it a way of protesting against aspects of your work that you don't enjoy, a means of making excuses for doing a less than satisfactory job or a need to manipulate and create crisis situations? Only you can analyze your problems and decide what they really are. But make sure you don't omit this crucial step.

## *Goals and Alternatives*

The purpose of this whole process is to generate goals that you can use to make decisions and solve problems. This is the time to determine what you are really trying to accomplish — eliminate paperwork, get it done on time, do it more completely, feel less pressured, resentful or manipulated? By now you should be able to identify a real problem and a true goal.

Now start brainstorming. Think of as many possible ways as you can to reach your goal. Don't be concerned with reality, practicality or feasibility at this stage; just try to generate as many solutions as you can. The idea is to get away from your usual way of looking at problems and to try to come up with new and creative approaches. The longer the list, the more possibilities you will have to choose from.

For example, let's assume that you have determined your true goal:

> Documentation will be done on time and will meet acceptable professional standards.

A list of possible strategies might look like this —

- Hire a secretary
- Do a little writing every day
- Take a course in writing
- Devote a large chunk of time only to documentation
- Hire a consultant
- Buy new pens

51

- Do it with someone else
- Write on the beach
- Buy a book with examples
- Change locations
- Play music in the background
- Find someone else to do it
- Do it first thing in the morning
- Get new forms
- Change the regulations
- Buy a dictionary
- Do it last thing before going home
- Do paperwork instead of eating lunch
- Reward yourself after each one completed
- Have someone else evaluate your work
- Do rough copy, have someone else enter in charts
- Keep daily notes on residents
- Set up new system
- Get input from other staff members
- Practice on imaginary residents
- Read other people's notes
- Alternate with more pleasant tasks

From this list it should be possible to come up with at least a few promising solutions. These still should be just general ideas. Don't worry about implementation. That comes later. Cross out those that are obviously bad ideas or definitely impossible to implement. But don't be too hasty. Make sure that you have explored all the alternatives and that they really are implausible. Consider those that you have tried before and see if you can determine ways to change them so that they might be tried again more successfully.

Pick out the most promising ones and see if they can be combined to make a still more effective solution. Explore the possible consequences of each course of action. Will others be affected? What might their reactions be? Will the effects be short or long term? Will they be more positive than negative?

Ask yourself "What would happen if ...?" when weighing alternatives or trying to reach a decision. It can be helpful to make a list of positive and negative consequences for each possibility, particularly when choosing between a limited number of alternatives. For example, in trying to decide whether to take a newly offered job or to stay in your present facility, you might have a list that looks something like this —

| Old Job | New Job |
|---|---|
| Positive<br>• Friendships<br>• Shorter commute<br>• Small, friendly, privately owned facility<br>• Flexible working hours | Positive<br>• More money<br>• Promotion<br>• Meeting new people<br>• More room for advancement |
| Negative<br>• Less money<br>• Less prestige<br>• Limited opportunities for advancement | Negative<br>• Longer commute<br>• Leaving friends<br>• Leaving residents<br>• Big, impersonal, corporation<br>• Pre-determined working hours |

Only you can weigh the factors in terms of their importance to you, but it should be helpful to see the trade-off in black and white.

# *Action*

Now is the time to think about the specifics. Look at your list of possible strategies and select those that look promising and could possibly be implemented. Your decision should be directed toward reaching the goal and solving the problem and should be based on good judgment and realistic evaluation of the alternatives.

Use the list that was developed to meet the goal:

> Documentation will be done on time and will meet acceptable professional standards.

Things that might meet the criteria are underlined.

- Hire a secretary
- Do a little writing everyday
- Take a course in writing
- Devote a large chunk of time only to documentation
- Hire a consultant
- Buy new pens
- Do it with someone else
- Write on the beach
- Buy a book with examples
- Change locations
- Play music in the background
- Find someone else to do it
- Do it first thing in the morning
- Get new forms
- Change the regulations
- Buy a dictionary
- Do it last thing before going home
- Do paperwork instead of eating lunch
- Reward yourself after each one completed

- Have someone else evaluate your work
- Do rough copy, have someone else enter in charts
- Keep daily notes on residents
- Set up new system
- Get input from other staff members
- Practice on imaginary residents
- Read other people's notes
- Alternate with more pleasant tasks

But before you can decide which to implement, you need more information. The first step might be to go to your administrator. Tell him/her that you are aware of your problem, committed to doing something about it and would like to find out if there is any help available. Are there funds for buying books, attending courses or workshops, hiring a consultant? Are there secretarial services that you could use or others that could help with some of your duties until you get caught up?

If the answer is "no" to all of these, then you must decide if you are able and/or willing to pay for some of them yourself. If so, you must choose those which appear to be most valuable. If you are not, then eliminate them from your list and look at the others you selected that do not require expenditures.

Perhaps now you will review your working hours, activities schedule, locations where you presently do documentation and other personnel in the facility who might be able to help you. As you continue through this process, you will refine the list until you are left with the strategies can be implemented.

Next comes the actual design of an action plan. Consider the consequences that you have identified and the people that will be affected. Consult with them and then outline steps, time frames and deadlines. Here is a possible action plan.

- After the completion of each activity, I will set aside five minutes to jot down notes on residents that might be helpful in writing updates.

- I will not leave the facility any night until I have satisfactorily completed two quarterly updates. (After I am caught up, this will be reduced to one.)

- Every Friday at 3 PM, I will meet with the social worker, discuss new residents and review the documentation that we have completed that week.

# Evaluate the Results

Evaluation is the last step in problem-solving. Is the plan working? Have the proper strategies been selected? Are you following through? Make sure that you don't confuse lack of effectiveness of the plan with your negligence in implementing it. But, if you haven't implemented it, why not? Is it impractical or have you attacked the wrong problem? If necessary, go through the process again until you have identified the real problem and created useful solutions.

If it is working, evaluate how well and whether more strategies may be needed to make it even more effective. What are your time frames? Is this a short- or long-term solution? If it has not ceased to be a problem or if you have made the wrong decision, where do you go from here?

Most problems can be solved if attacked in this fashion. However, new ones will undoubtedly take their place and you will have the opportunity to use this technique again and again.

## Pitfalls to Avoid

A word of caution is necessary to help you avoid some common mistakes. Use of the processes mentioned here should prove helpful.

1. Don't worry about decisions already made. Once you decide on an action, do it decisively. Don't go over the same ground and think that perhaps you made the wrong choice. Perhaps you did, but it has been done and you will do better next time.

2. Don't re-invent the wheel. Use your own experience and that of others. If it has worked in the past, chances are that it will again.

3. Don't make a big deal out of everything, even minor decisions. Some things simply do not require a great amount of time and effort and might better be ignored.

4. Don't stick your finger in every pie. Your input is not always necessary (or welcome) in every decision and problem-solving situation.

5. Do admit it when you've made a wrong decision. Nobody is perfect. Don't compound your mistakes by pretending to be perfect or by blaming someone else.

6. Consult with others who might be affected by decisions or solutions. If they are part of the problem, they deserve to be consulted concerning its resolution.

7. Don't promise things you can't deliver and make decisions where follow-through is impossible. Some options may seem to be the most desirable, but if they are not feasible in your particular situation, they are not really options.

## Chapter 6

# How to Recognize and Handle Stress

*Are there mornings when you have trouble getting up and to work on time?*

*Are there times when you feel overwhelmed and have difficulty coping?*

*Do you often suffer from headaches, appetite changes, irritability or butterflies in your stomach?*

It could be that you are being exposed to an unusually high level of stress. You may need some help in the management of stress.

"Stress" has become a very "in" term and one that we read about constantly. But what exactly is *stress*? By definition, it is physical, mental or emotional strain or tension that disrupts a person's equilibrium.

Chronic stress can affect people in many different ways. For convenience, these can be divided into three major categories:

1. Physiological — can affect every system of the body and be a contributing factor in many diseases, including high blood pressure, stroke, headaches, back pain, ulcers, digestive or respiratory disorders;

2. Emotional — feelings of being threatened, overwhelmed, anxious, angry, helpless, depressed or guilty;

3. Potentially self-destructive habits — drug and alcohol abuse, smoking, over- or under-eating, inability to sleep or sleeping excessively.

Everybody, at certain times in their lives, experiences high levels of stress and its accompanying symptoms. Indeed, a certain amount of stress is necessary for a useful existence. Although complete absence of stress leads to boredom and dissatisfaction, high levels of continuing stress are undesirable and in many cases, even dangerous.

## Causes of Stress

Unfortunately, the very qualities that lead people to choose a helping profession such as an activity professional, are quite possibly the same ones that make them more vulnerable to high levels of stress. These people often are sensitive, with high ideals, great enthusiasm and a desire to be useful and needed.

In addition, many aspects inherent in the job of activity professional also contribute to stress. You are probably only too familiar with most of these, but let's look at them a little more closely and identify why they create stress.

First, the issue of isolation. Many activity professionals are alone in their facilities. They have no one else there who understands exactly what they do and nobody with whom they can test ideas. This can lead to feelings of loneliness and uncertainty.

Closely allied to this is the poorly defined role that often accompanies this occupation. Most activity professionals have very limited (or no) input into their job description. They may lack clear guidelines for performance, receive inadequate or poor training for their jobs and have little supervision. In many cases, they are called upon to make a large number of decisions without preparation or support.

In addition, they often are or feel that they are, not really appreciated and held in low esteem by others in the facility and in the community. The lack of clear identity leads to feelings of inferiority and powerlessness. And these lead to stress.

So do the demands and expectations that go with the job. Many activity professionals try to be all things to all people. They are hard-pressed to meet the expectations of both the residents and the administration, to say nothing of their own expectations. They may feel that they are the victims of divided loyalties and can't possibly fulfill all the conflicting demands of the job. Thus, they cannot complete the large amounts of required paperwork, meet individual resident needs, satisfy their administrators and still maintain their schedules. Often there is a great deal of resentment at a job that demands working nights and weekends and a great deal of guilt about that resentment and about the things that don't get done. That guilt is a combination of anxiety and anger towards themselves and others.

Another source of stress is the limited mobility that usually accompanies the job of activity professional. There are few opportunities for promotion within their organizations. And this is accompanied by low salaries and a lack of means of measuring on-the-job success. People work for a variety of reasons, but need to get personal satisfaction from the job as well as recognition, rewards and a sense of working towards a goal. Unfortunately, many good people leave this field every year. They feel that they have accomplished all that they possibly can within the confines of their particular job and there is just no place else to go as an activity director.

Yet another potential source of stress is the difficulty experienced in separating work from personal life. Balancing all of the roles that most people fill is not easy at best, but when one's job is very emotionally demanding, it often seems impossible. It is sometimes equally impossible to leave personal problems behind when one comes to work.

Relationships can also contribute to stress. Many people find themselves in the position of spending almost all their time socializing with their co-workers, which makes it almost impossible to avoid talking and thinking about work-related concerns. Others, in trying not to get caught up in this, find that they may have difficulties with some people who think they are avoiding them. When a co-worker is put in a position of suddenly supervising a colleague, problems can arise, as they can from many other supervisory-subordinate situations. Inability to plan effectively, manage time or delegate authority and lack of training in supervisory skills all can be contributing factors to stress.

Stress is due to an accumulation of factors that are operating at the same time. It is rarely the result of one isolated cause.

## Coping with Stress

To begin with, you must recognize that there are stressors in your life and acknowledge their existence. Then try to identify the sources. To help in this process, you might ask yourself:

- Are there certain things that always provoke stress in me, such as high noise levels, certain people, situations such as speaking in public?
- Are there times when I am more likely to feel stress and do I recognize them?
- Do I continually put myself in a position where I feel a lack of control or overload?
- Is pressure a necessary part of my work or is it occurring as a result of the way that I handle my job?
- What am I doing to make situations more stressful than they need to be?
- Am I meeting some of my needs by maintaining this stress level? What am I getting out of it?
- What else is going on in my life that is also contributing to my stress?

There are a number of life events that are considered highly stressful in themselves. These may include changes in marital situations, living arrangements, employment, finances, children leaving home, deaths of close friends or relatives or anything else that impacts your daily routine. When these are combined with minor hassles and pressures, stress levels rise accordingly.

The next step in dealing effectively with stress is to recognize how you react to it. There are vast differences in stress thresholds and individual reactions. What is only a minor annoyance to one person may be a major catastrophe to someone else. Different personality types interpret events differently.

If you are unaware of how you react to stress or want to get a clearer picture, ask your family or those close to you. You will probably be amazed how accurately they can identify the things that you react to and the ways in which you react.

(But make sure that their honesty is not going to add further stress!)

Do you usually recognize what your body is trying to tell you? Headaches, stomach upsets, muscle ache between the shoulders, etc. often are the signs that the body's defense system has been called into play. If they are ignored, it can become dangerous. The defense system may no longer be able to handle the stress and some kind of breakdown may occur.

Are some of your responses self-destructive or self-defeating? Things like over-indulgences in food or drink, temper tantrums, extravagant purchases or naps to avoid action can all be stress responses. Are you aware of when and why you react in this way? And, do these responses help you to cope successfully or do they add further to your stress level, often compounding it with guilt?

What are you doing now that works and what else could you be doing? This brings us to the last step in this process and that is to develop a stress management program that *works for you.*

Stated most simply, there are two major ways of handling stress — eliminate the source or learn to handle it better. Let's look first at eliminating the source. Take the list of stressors that you have identified and see if you can effectively rid yourself of some of them. Are there people you don't have to see as frequently, jobs you can delegate to others, different ways of doing things, different times, different travel routes, different locations. Look at some of the items on that list and ask why you react to them the way that you do. What in the situation or about the person causes that reaction in you? Can you eliminate it or learn to deal with it better?

How much are you willing to risk? This is an essential question when you begin to evaluate your stressors. Learn to ask yourself, "What will happen if ...?" And, are you willing to take that chance?

If you decide to take action, don't put it off indefinitely. Choose your fights carefully. But once you decide to take a stand, choose a course of action and follow it. Often the mere act of reaching a decision helps, but stress will begin to rise again if you allow the situation to persist.

If you are not willing or able to take the risk to eliminate the stress, that leaves you with the second alternative, learning to handle it better. Generally, in order to do this, you must make some changes in the way you handle your life. Define your own needs. What do you need to get out of or eliminate from, stressful situations? Learn to talk up and define these needs better — and the feelings you have about them — to other people. Ask them to share their expectations with you so you will understand them better and have a better feel for what your role should be.

Try to become better organized: make plans, set deadlines, delegate tasks. Learn to say "no" when it's appropriate. If you have a choice, don't overburden yourself with more than you can handle. Make compromises. Recognize and accept your limitations. Define your priorities.

Identify other people with whom you can share your concerns and feelings. Take time out when you feel overwhelmed and change tasks, locations or associates.

For those things that are unavoidable, try to work them into your schedule at times when you are best able to handle them. Unpleasant tasks become less so if they are worked into your routine and are bracketed by others that are more pleasurable.

Learn to reward yourself for minor accomplishments and to consider your own needs in situations. Find other sources of success and satisfaction so that you are not dependent on only your job or other people's view of you.

Use humor and learn to laugh at yourself. Avoid self-medications and excessive amounts of caffeine, alcohol, tobacco and food. Try to balance your life and relieve tension with sufficient periods of exercise, work, fun, sleep and just plain loafing.

## Stress Management Techniques

In addition to these suggestions, there are a number of strategies that have been identified as being useful in the management of stress. Of course, not all will work for everyone, but from among the following list, you should be able to select one or more that might do it for you.

1. Learn and practice effective time management techniques.

2. Find someone to give you a neck and shoulder massage.

3. Listen to your body. The technique of biofeedback is one of the most effective means of dealing with stress. By recognizing the symptoms, people can be taught to control pulse, blood pressure, headaches, allergic reactions, etc. Consult your physician and see if this is something that you could learn to do.

4. Relaxation exercises. There are a variety of these that bring good results such as deep breathing and progressive

relaxation which entails consciously relaxing one group of muscles at a time.

5. Mental imagery. When faced with an unpleasant situation, remove yourself. For example, imagine you are on a beach. Try to involve all your senses: smell the salt water and suntan lotion, feel the sun and the sand, hear the surf and the seagulls, etc. If people intimidate you, picture them in a situation where they are not so threatening, perhaps without any clothes. If you are in a position where you feel inadequate, picture yourself as masterful and in charge.

6. "What's the worst thing that could happen?" routine. If you find yourself in a situation where your stress level is rising and there is nothing you can do, try this technique. Suppose you are caught in a traffic jam and you know you are going to miss an important appointment. What can possibly happen? Will someone be angry at you? Will you miss an opportunity? Will you be able to explain or re-schedule? And the second part is "What will I do then?" The act of looking at possible consequences instead of dealing with nameless fears helps to put situations into perspective and makes coping with them much simpler.

7. Exercise. Almost any regular rhythmic exercise will do. Walking, jogging, biking, swimming, aerobics, dancing — any or all of these will allow for a break in tension and are an effective means of ridding yourself of stored up anxieties.

## Chapter 7

# How to Work with a Consultant

*"By the way," said the administrator to the activity director, "You are getting a consultant. She will be here next Tuesday at ten o'clock to meet with you."*

For many of you, this may be the way that you first hear that you are going to be working with a consultant. Whatever the reason — your not being fully qualified, your corporation employing a consultant or a state surveyor "suggesting" that some help is needed — the reaction will probably be the same.

"What is a consultant? What can s/he do for me? How does a consultant operate? What is my responsibility in a consultancy relationship?" Not knowing what to expect, you may feel very threatened. Who needs someone coming in who may rate you and your program poorly? You might even lose your job!

## What is a Consultant?

A consultant is one who gives professional advice. S/he provides knowledge and experience to help produce a solution to a problem or to outline a course of action to be taken.

Consultants provide guidance so that others may do their jobs more effectively.

Consultants usually remain removed from direct services but do deal with those factors that influence all the residents in the facility. However, in some situations, activity consultation may differ from the classical definition and the consultant may also be expected to work directly with the residents.

A list of desirable qualities for an activity consultant might include the abilities to:

- clarify and convey what the role of the consultant is and what s/he expects from you
- deal effectively with individuals and groups
- remain objective
- stay on task
- deal with resistance
- listen effectively
- give skillful and meaningful feedback
- respect confidentiality
- separate problem identification from problem solution
- help in evaluating alternatives that will be satisfying to those directly involved

Additionally, activity consultants should have knowledge of and be familiar with:

- the regulations affecting the type of facility you work in, particularly activity programming
- psychology, physiology and medical conditions that have implications for activity participation
- particular activities that can be used to effectively meet identified individual needs of residents

- methods of determining if the program is effective in covering the spiritual, physical, intellectual, social, work and creative needs of all residents
- activity analysis which is the method that is used to break down activities and determine their methods, safety factors, mental and physical demands, equipment and supplies required, appropriate teaching approaches and suitability for individual residents

Effective consultants —

1. involve the activity professionals in as much of the planning as possible by letting them set priorities and determine the areas in which the consultant can be of most value.

2. recognize the normal concerns of the consultee and, therefore, provide complete information to prevent rumors and speculation.

3. should also be aware of the importance of group habits and norms and not suggest changes that would interfere with working hours, lunch and break times or commuting schedules, if at all possible.

Consultation is a very special relationship. Although the consultant may have specialized knowledge in a given field, all parties are considered of equal rank and status. A consultant may provide advice, information or education, but the consultee is always free to accept or reject it.

Another unique characteristic of this relationship is that the consultant is usually an outsider. This can be both an advantage and a disadvantage. Although it may provide a fresh unbiased point of view, it does not allow for the intimate knowledge of the residents, staff, organization, etc. that may be necessary to grasp situations in their entirety.

Consultants to an activity program primarily should be considered as agents of change or as facilitators whose roles are to evaluate the program, change the focus if necessary, help in identifying problems and solutions and serve as resource persons.

## *What Can a Consultant Do for Me?*

The personnel of every facility, both administrative and activities, have differing ideas of the function and scope of the consultant's role. Therefore, it is imperative that these be discussed in the beginning of the relationship so that everyone will have the same expectations, the same ideas of the general direction that the consultation will take and perhaps, even to determine if the consultant is the right person for this particular job. In order to have a good working relationship, everyone must be working from the same agenda.

Assessment and evaluation are among the prime functions that activity consultants normally provide. In fact, they will probably devote the first several sessions to finding out as much as possible about your facility. Specifically, they must familiarize themselves with:

1. Resident population: numbers, levels of care, ages, diagnoses, predominant ethnic and religious groups

2.  Administration: attitudes toward activity programming, personnel and having a consultant; commitment to change and education; lines of authority

3.  Activity set-up and personnel: rooms available for programs, scheduling programs, storage, budget, attitudes, experience and training of personnel

4.  Activity programming: scope, consideration of individual resident needs and interests, group and individual activities, night and weekend coverage, utilization of volunteers and community resources, communication and publicity

5.  Documentation of services: meeting requirements, effective and efficient procedures

6.  Other departments: support, communication and cooperation between them; acceptance of necessity and desirability of activities

Consultants also serve as sounding boards. They hear grievances and test new ideas. Because they are outsiders and do not have as much at stake, they can often make administration aware of problems that the activity professional cannot. Through the use of their consultation reports and formal or informal discussions, they can serve as intermediaries. Not only can they make administration aware of identified problems, they may also serve this function with some of the regulatory agencies, helping to clarify for them why things are done or not done a certain way. Or they may advise the agencies of problems in implementing programs of which the agencies may not be aware.

Consultants should be familiar with all pertinent regulations and be able to interpret them and advise about how they can best be implemented. They should be able to provide you with documentation training. They will review what is currently being done and suggest ways to streamline procedures, make forms more efficient and, if necessary, improve the content and effectiveness of the notes themselves.

They should also serve as resource persons. They are able to provide information on available community resources, helpful publications, workshops and seminars, sources of specialized help and exactly what is out there that might help you make your activity department function more effectively.

Consultants can also demonstrate how theories can be put into practice — relating principles of activity programming to the everyday functioning of your department and its program and applying motivational techniques for stimulating and sustaining resident interest. They can advise about volunteer programs — determine needs, suggest possible sources, develop programs for training and orientation and suggest ways that your volunteer program could be improved.

Consultants should be skilled in working with you to solve problems. Their role is not to tell you how to do things, but rather to help you clarify situations and evaluate alternatives. They should be able to teach problem-solving techniques and show how they can be used by you in present and future situations.

They can also help you develop a philosophy for the activity department in order to help you determine its exact function within the facility, its long-range goals and objectives. They can support the development of a policies and procedures manual, providing samples and suggestions. They can advise about scheduling and efficient use of personnel time. They can also suggest new techniques and activities to broaden the scope of the program and to more effectively meet individual identified needs and interests, as well as activity adaptations that might be useful with particular residents.

Most consultants recognize that they have responsibility to the total facility and not just to your specific department. To this end, consultants of all the departments should meet to coordinate their goals and policies and to ensure that they are all working towards the same objectives.

They can also provide other services to the total facility, such as in-service or continuing education programs — not only to help explain the function and importance of activity but, depending on their field of expertise, in other areas as well. They can bring to administrative and other staff any changes in regulations that may impact activity programming, as well as suggesting means of implementing change that may make the programming more effective. They can advise about appropriate staffing requirements, equipment storage space, best use of space for activity implementation and activities that could be added to make the program more effective. They can also serve on facility committees and be involved in setting resident care policies, particularly in the area of activities.

## How Does a Consultant Operate?

What can you expect from a typical visit? Consultants, like all people, have their own style. Some spend most of their time in discussion and problem-solving. Others will observe activities and critique them afterwards. Or, they may prefer to lead the activity themselves and have you observe. Some will suggest readings and talk about them on their next visit. Others will give you case histories and ask you to come up with solutions. They may suggest visits to other facilities to see what types of programs they have or encourage you to attend workshops or seminars in areas that they think may prove helpful. Sometimes they will ask you to do tasks which will then be reviewed and evaluated. Any or all of these are possible ways for a consultant to operate. All have validity and by no means do these represent all the possibilities.

## What Can't a Consultant Do For Me?

Consultants can't actually implement change; they can only advise and suggest. Because of this advisory capacity, they have no real authority within the system. They do not have any responsibility for carrying out programs or suggested changes.

They cannot be aware of all the facets of the organization and must rely a great deal on your input to get a real feeling for the dynamics that are operating. Without this and the communication of your needs and priorities, it is difficult for them, in the limited time they are usually in the facility, to get a clear picture. Therefore, the more information you give them, the better able they will be to satisfy your needs.

Consultants, no matter how skilled, cannot be expected to overcome your inertia or resistance to change. They can work with you only as much as you allow. Certainly, some feelings of defensiveness and anxiety are normal, but if you are not willing to meet them at least halfway, consultants cannot help you overcome those roadblocks. Much valuable time is wasted and sometimes nothing gets accomplished, because of the resentment or the hurt pride of the activity professionals.

Consultants cannot interfere in the workings of other departments that are outside the legitimate scope of their sanction. Although they may be able to identify problems that exist, they can only get involved when they impact upon activities. And, even then, there is definitely a limit to where they are allowed to intercede.

No consultant can be expected to have all the answers and solutions. They usually have built up a good framework of references, experiences and experts to whom they can turn for guidance, but may not have the answer immediately when the problem is raised. But they should be able to, at least, point you in the right direction and introduce methods that might help you find the answers yourself.

## What is My Responsibility?

It is not the total responsibility of the consultant to determine the course and outcomes of the consultancy. You also play a major role in this process.

The scheduling of meetings is the activity director's responsibility. Certainly these should be planned for a time that is mutually convenient but, most importantly, at a time when you can arrange for coverage of scheduled activities by someone else. Consultants should never just "drop in" and expect that time will immediately become available to them. This is acceptable only if they have come to observe, and even then it is questionable whether prior notice is required or not. The place selected to hold the consultation should be private and quiet and not where you will be constantly interrupted by phone calls and visitors.

Inform the administrator of the consultant's impending visit and determine is s/he wishes to see him/her or pass on any message. Although consultants usually include the date and time of their next visit in their report, it is a courtesy to inform the administrator and helpful to both of them.

You should take time to orient consultants to the facility. Take them on a guided tour, make them feel welcome, provide a safe place where they may store their belongings, make provisions for lunch, if necessary, and introduce them to other staff members so that the legitimacy of their role is established.

Be prepared for the consultant's visit. Set up an agenda, if it was not established at the last meeting. Get in the habit of jotting down questions, problems, things that arise between visits. It is entirely appropriate to call consultants to ask them to bring resource material on a particular subject or to suggest that there is something that you would like them to be prepared to discuss. If you are asked to complete an assignment for the next visit, make sure that it is finished and available for review.

Help to clarify your expectations and how, in your opinion, consultants can help you. Do you, indeed, have the same set of expectations and the same agenda? If they don't bring it up, make sure that you do. Make an effort to get in touch with your own attitudes, prejudices and needs in this relationship and try to make sure that you are reacting appropriately and to the right things. Do you have a sincere desire to change existing conditions and eliminate problems? Are you open-minded to suggestions that the consultant might make? Or are you coming up with 101 reasons why they won't work?

Help with the assessment and evaluation. Give the consultant as much information as you possibly can. That doesn't mean gossip, rumor or personality profiles, but a sincere evaluation of how the facility works, some of the problems you have identified and some of the positive resources that you have to call upon. Don't expect quick results, but do outline long-term goals and work towards them.

Be prepared for termination of the consultancy. Don't become overly dependent on your consultant. Good consultants work themselves out of jobs and should be judged by how well the consultees carry on after they leave, using the knowledge and skills they have gained. Work toward this end. Most consultants remain available for questions by telephone after they leave, but don't overdo this or feel that you will be unable to continue once the consultants have left.

Don't ask them to compromise their loyalties. Often one of the most difficult problems for consultants is determining to whom they owe their allegiance. Although they are employed by the administration, they have a natural tendency to feel responsible to and for activity professionals with whom they are consulting. As all staff, they feel that the welfare of the residents is the paramount concern and may even feel an allegiance to the regulatory agencies which should be aware of situations that may be uncovered. It has sometimes been necessary for consultants to resign because situations observed and left unresolved have put them in a compromised position. If the situation involves resident abuse, the consultant (and every other person who witnesses the abuse, including you) is legally obligated to file a report with the appropriate state agency.

Most importantly, keep an open mind. Remember that consultants are there to help you. They are not there to judge you or to cost you your job, but rather to help you treat the residents more effectively.

Consultants have a responsibility in the relationship as well. They must be on time, prepared, willing to listen, ready to follow your lead and not armed with their own agenda.

As you can see, the success of a consultation relationship depends on many things — the skill of the consultant, the expectations of all concerned and perhaps most importantly, your attitude and acceptance.

*Chapter 8*

# How to Improve Communication Skills

As you have seen from previous chapters, the most important set of skills that you need to be a true professional are those of effective communication. These are vital skills to the success of any organization and no person or program can function without them.

Communication is the means by which we express feelings, convey needs, resolve conflicts, give directions, clarify objectives and deal with people and groups. It is the process of giving and receiving information through the use of various devices, including symbols, gestures and voice intonations.

Communication has three parts and is not complete unless all three parts are involved — the sender, the message and the receiver.

## Types of Communication

The two major types of communication are written and verbal and both have advantages and disadvantages. The printed word is ideal for reaching large numbers of people and provides a permanent record of the communication. It also gives you an opportunity to carefully select words and rewrite if necessary. However, the biggest disadvantage is that it does not provide for feedback; that is, there is no way of knowing if the message that you sent is the one that was received. If the receiver does not understand or misinterprets the message, there are no immediate opportunities to correct these misconceptions. And, unfortunately, they sometimes can be acted upon before they can be cleared up.

On the other hand, verbal communication, while providing opportunities for immediate feedback also provides opportunities for greater misunderstanding. It is dependent on the receiver's ability to listen effectively, which, as you will see, is often a problem in itself. Verbal communication is, no doubt, faster but does not allow the sender to consider his words and message as carefully. This, too, can be a negative factor.

Sometimes a combination of both methods is the most effective means of communication, i.e. an oral message followed by a memo that repeats and reinforces what was said. This allows both parties to make sure that they have the same understanding of the matter at hand.

There are also many other ways that people communicate. Body language can be very effective in conveying messages. Gestures, movements, mannerisms, bearing and facial expressions all add immeasurably to the communication process. Think how much can be said with a frown, smile, wink or grimace of distaste. And, what kind of message do we get from someone who is blushing, perspiring profusely, trembling or crying? How significant to the communication is the way people touch one another (for example, the firm handshake) and the amount or lack of eye contact?

It is important, however, to always consider body language in terms of its agreement with the words that are being said. The gestures themselves only have significance as part of a total picture. What does it mean when someone is paying a compliment without eye contact and while shuffling papers? What message is being sent when a person puts his/her arm around another that s/he is criticizing? Is the action in agreement with the words? Are you aware of the non-verbal behaviors that you use? Are they distracting or do they help to reinforce the message that you are trying to send?

Another type of communication is the example that you set. Do you say one thing and do another? Do you suggest standards for dress, manners, responses and respect for others that are actually quite different from what you, yourself, do? Which message do you think is being received?

We use other methods of non-verbal communication to send messages about ourselves. Our use of time is one method, for instance. Being consistently early, on time or late each makes a definite statement. Our style of dress, the design of our personal environments and how we set up work areas to designate rank all communicate information about us.

There are recognized cultural differences in the ways that people use space. Some people feel very threatened if others get too close or infringe on what they feel to be their territory. We are conditioned from an early age to know the appropriate distance to keep and exactly how long we can look at someone we are passing without having to look away. Can you remember times when you have felt uncomfortable because someone held your eye too long or came uncomfortably close?

Some communicators use this to their advantage when the situation is appropriate. But be aware of the dynamics that are operating and try to assess how others are reacting to your presence in their space.

## Communication Problems

Many communication problems arise because people are different. Even when looking at the same thing, they do not experience and interpret it in the same way. We are taught what to see and hear and events we have not experienced before sometimes make no sense to us. It takes successive experiences to finally recognize a sequence or pattern that is meaningful. And when we try to relay this to someone else who has had different experiences, we often run into difficulties. Have you ever told a friend something funny that happened to you and gotten very little response? Often, we get out of it by saying, "Well, I guess you had to be there." But even if they had, their reaction probably would still not have been the same as yours!

Words must be carefully chosen and clearly defined. There are over 600,000 words in the English language with more being added all the time. Most of us use about 2,000 in our daily conversations and the 500 most commonly used words have about 14,000 definitions between them.

One simple example of this is the word "fast." If I were to say "Make it fast," you might think that you had better hurry. But I might mean to tie it up, as in making a boat fast or to make sure that the color doesn't run as in being color fast. From a religious standpoint, to fast means to abstain, but ... a "fast" woman abstains from nothing! So, as you can see, you cannot always be sure the words you use are conveying the message that you intended. Many communication problems result from the assumption that everyone knows what you are talking about and that you know what others are talking about.

Some causes of problems include the tendencies of listeners to:

- be defensive, close-minded or resistant to change
- be distracted by their own personal concerns
- jump to conclusions, finishing the speaker's message with their own thoughts and expectations — this is called wishful hearing, i.e. hearing what you want to hear
- dislike or have personal prejudice toward the speaker, perhaps because of status differences or past experiences
- think ahead about what they want to respond when it is their turn to speak
- lack interest or concentration

Problems that are attributable to the sender of messages include:

- tendency to talk before thinking, to ramble and be disorganized
- poor speaking habits, including monotonous tone, use of clichés, jargon or irritating verbal mannerisms (such as the infamous "you know" scattered frequently throughout)
- use of a style that is offensive to the listener, such as threatening, preaching, interrogating, humoring, blaming, lecturing, criticizing or commanding

The biggest block to communication is people's inability to listen to each other intelligently, with understanding and skill. How a message is interpreted depends on the listener's physiological and psychological state at the time. Listeners may be inclined to censor and filter information according to their own value system but not let the speaker know that there is a difficulty in understanding. In short, few people know how to listen effectively.

As we've established, a message hasn't been communicated if it is sent over an open circuit. It is only complete if another has listened and understood it. But listening is hard work and not just a passive and automatic response. Your brain is capable of processing information at a rate four to five times faster than people can speak, so it requires great concentration to prevent your mind from wandering when it is not fully engaged.

Effective listening can be learned. However, it is dependent on your ability to empathize and identify with someone else's viewpoint. This doesn't mean you have to agree, but a good listener must attempt to understand what the speaker is trying to convey. It is perfectly permissible *after* you have listened, to counter with your own point of view.

The most common barrier to listening is talking. In order to have good communication, it is necessary to curb your own need to talk and give others a chance. And this means really listening to the words being used as well as the non-verbal clues. It also means listening to subordinates with the same courtesy as you show to your supervisors and not blocking communication attempts with small talk or your own agenda.

## *Improving Your Communication Skills*

People who have the desire to improve their communication skills can do so with practice. Here are some guidelines and suggestions that might help:

- Get feedback from others concerning what they think your skill level of verbal and written communication is. Don't be defensive about their criticisms. Try to learn from them.
- If possible, tape some of your conversational sessions and try to evaluate yourself objectively.
- Listen to others whose communication skills you admire and try to determine what makes them effective communicators.
- Learn to organize your thoughts in any conversation before you begin to speak and stick to the purpose you have identified.
- Try to minimize distractions when communicating; give speaking and listening your total concentration.
- Try to identify and start with your listener's concerns.
- Try to see other people's point of view even if you don't like them or agree with them.
- Be prepared and totally familiar with information that you are trying to relay to others.
- Don't be afraid to say "I don't think I understood that. Could you explain it again?"
- Encourage and allow time for feedback so you can be certain that others understand you.
- Develop an efficient system of communication within your facility that works for you.
- Take every opportunity to speak in public before small and large groups until you feel comfortable doing so.
- Talk less and listen more.

And, finally, remember that communication is going on all the time. Try to be aware of the messages you are sending when you don't think that you are sending any. Check to see if you are being perceived by others in the fashion that you intend. And listen closely so that you can better interpret those with whom you are communicating.

# A Final Word

By this time, it should be evident that none of the skills outlined in this manual come easily to most of us. However, with motivation and practice they can be developed and constantly improved. I hope this "survival" guide will serve as an inspiration and starting point. The rest is up to you.

# Bibliography and Suggested Readings

American Health Care Association. *Standards for Activity Coordinators and Activity Programming in Long-Term Care Facilities.* (Pamphlet).

Anderson, John. "Giving and Receiving Feedback." *Personnel Administration*, March-April, 1968.

Baker, John K. & Robert H. Schaffer. "Making Staff Consulting More Effective." *Harvard Business Review.* January-February, 1969.

Best Martini, Elizabeth, Mary Anne Weeks and Priscilla Wirth. 1996. **Long Term Care for Activity and Social Service Professionals**. Ravensdale, WA: Idyll Arbor, Inc.

Blanchard, Kenneth & Spencer Johnson. 1982. **The One Minute Manager**. New York: William Morrow & Co., Inc.

Boyd, David P. & David E. Gumpert. "Coping With Entrepreneurial Stress." *Harvard Business Review.* March-April, 1983.

Carroll, Kathy, Ed. 1978. **Social Behaviors and Relationships**. Minneapolis, MN: Ebenezer Center for Aging and Human Development.

Charlotte, Dr. Lu, June, 1983. "Professionalism" Keynote
Address. Southern California Conference of Activity
Coordinators.

Cunninghis, Richelle N. 1995. **Reality Activities: A How To
Manual for Increasing Orientation, Second Edition**.
Ravensdale, WA: Idyll Arbor, Inc.

Cunninghis, Richelle N. and Elizabeth Best Martini. 1996.
**Quality Assurance for Activity Programs, Second
Edition**. Ravensdale, WA: Idyll Arbor, Inc.

D'Antonio-Nocera, Anne, Nancy DeBolt, and Nadine Touhey,
Eds. 1996. **The Professional Activity Manager and
Consultant**. Ravensdale, WA: Idyll Arbor, Inc.

Davis, Martha, Elizabeth Robbins Eshelman and Matthew
McKay. 1995. **The Relaxation and Stress Reduction
Workbook, Fourth Edition**. Oakland, CA: New
Harbinger Publications, Inc.

Department of Health, Education and Welfare, Draft
September 8, 1972. **Planner's and Instructor's Guide for
Activities Coordinators Continuing Education Programs**.

Fabun, Don. 1968. **Communications: The Transfer of
Meaning**. Beverly Hills: Glencoe Press.

FallCreek, Stephanie & Molly Mettler. 1982. **A Healthy Old
Age: A Sourcebook for Health Promotion With Older
Adults.** Baltimore, MD: U.S. Department of Health and
Human Services.

Fish, Harriet U. 1971. **Activities Programs for Senior
Citizens**. West Nyack, NY: Parker Publishing Co.

Haimann, Theo & Raymond L. Hilgert. 1977. **Supervision: Concepts and Practices of Management**. Cincinnati: South-Western Publishing Co.

Hausser, D. L., P. A. Pecorella, & A. L. Webster. 1977. **Survey-Guided Development II: A Manual for Consultants**. La Jolla: University Associates, Inc.

Holdeman, Elizabeth. 1979. **A Guide for the Activity Coordinator in a Skilled Nursing Facility**. Sacramento: California Department of Health Services.

Jennings, Eugene E. 1960. **An Anatomy of Leadership: Princes, Heroes and Superman**. New York: McGraw Hill.

Lakein, Alan. 1974. **How to Get Control of Your Time and Your Life**. New York: Signet Books.

Livingston, Frances M. & Nadine B. O'Sullivan, Eds. 1977. **Occupational Therapy Consultancy in the Skilled Nursing Facility, An Overview**. Southern California Occupational Therapy Consultants Group.

McKay, Matthew, Martha Davis, and Patrick Fanning. 1981. **Thoughts and Feelings: The Art of Cognitive Stress Intervention**. Oakland, Ca: New Harbinger Publications.

McKay, Matthew, Martha Davis, and Patrick Fanning. 1995. **Messages: The Communication Skills Book, Second Edition**. Oakland, Ca: New Harbinger Publications.

Metropolitan New York District, New York State Occupational Therapy Association, February 26-27, 1971. *Report of an Institute. The Occupational Therapist Consultant in Nursing Homes*.

91

Mial, H. Curtis. "What is a Consultant?" Reprint from *Public Relations Journal,* November 1959.

Miller, Dulcy B. "Reflections Concerning an Activity Consultant by a Nursing Home Administrator." *The American Journal of Occupational Therapy.* Vol. 32. No. 6, July 1978.

Pines, Ayala & Ditsa Kafry. "Occupational Tedium in the Social Services." *Social Work.* Vol. 23. No. 6, November 1978.

Plachy, Roger. 1978. **When I Lead, Why Don't They Follow?** Chicago: Teach 'em, Inc.

Rue, Leslie W. & Lloyd Byars. 1982. **Supervision: Key Link to Productivity**. Homewood, IL: Richard D. Irwin, Inc.

Rutherford, Robert D. 1981. **Just In Time.** New York: John Wiley & Sons.

Scott, Dru. 1980. **How to Put More Time in Your Life**. New York: New American Library.

Selye, Hans. 1975. **Stress Without Distress**. New York: J. B. Lippincott.

Shuff, Frances and Joseph Kramer. "Organization Concepts, Part II Communication." *The American Journal of Occupational Therapy.* Vol. XXV. No. 8, 1971.

U.S. Department of Health, Education and Welfare, 1978. **Activities Coordinator's Guide**.

Wall, Nancy H. & Maureen Neistadt. 1982. **Stress**. Boston, MA: AIM for Health.